Absolute Beginner Series

Bed Yoga ~
Easy, Healing, Yoga Moves
You Can Do in Bed

by

Blythe Ayne, Ph.D.

Absolute Beginner Series

Bed Yoga ~
Easy, Healing, Yoga Moves You Can Do in Bed

by

Blythe Ayne, Ph.D.

Absolute Beginner Series
Bed Yoga -
Easy, Healing, Yoga Moves You Can Do in Bed
Blythe Ayne, Ph.D.

Emerson & Tilman, Publishers
129 Pendleton Way #55
Washougal, WA 98671

Bed Yoga -
Easy, Healing, Yoga Moves You Can Do in Bed

ebook ISBN: 978-1-947151-59-8
Paperback ISBN: 978-1-947151-60-4
Hardbound ISBN: 978-1-947151-61-1

[1. HEALTH & FITNESS / Yoga
2. HEALTH & FITNESS / Healing
3. BODY, MIND & SPIRIT / HEALING / Energy]

BIC: FM
First Edition

*Thank you with deep appreciation
to all my brilliant & kind manuscript avatars.*

DEDICATION:
Dedicated to all the amazing yoga instructors
I've had through the years
And to all yoga students, new and accomplished.
Every day, we are *Absolute Beginners*
With the beginner's mind of
Anticipation, Challenge, and Joy.

Table of Contents

Bed Yoga

The Poses

Why Bed Yoga?

There are a variety of reasons why you might discover bed yoga is right for you ....

Maybe you just woke up, and don't feel like hopping out of bed yet.

Perhaps you're under the weather and you're spending a couple days in bed.

Or you may be bedridden. Bed yoga is excellent for you! You'll exercise different muscle groups, gently in a healthy sequence.

It's a fact that going through yoga moves, if only in your mind's eye, causes your muscles to fire. So, let's fire up some muscles!

The softness or firmness of your mattress will have some bearing on the various *asana* (Sanskrit for "pose"), as will your own possible restriction of movement if dealing with an injury or other limitation. *This is your yoga!* Use the poses that you enjoy and that make your body feel happy, engaging in the movements the way that is best for you.

I love this about yoga—I never have to be perfect at it. Yoga does not have a mindset of competition. I always get to be an *Absolute Beginner*—and so do you!

One of my favorite yoga instructors, Richard Matusow, often starts his yoga class with *Shavasana*. When you're in bed, you're already in *Shavasana*!

A flower does not compete
With the flower next to it.
It just blooms.
Zen Shim

Shavasana

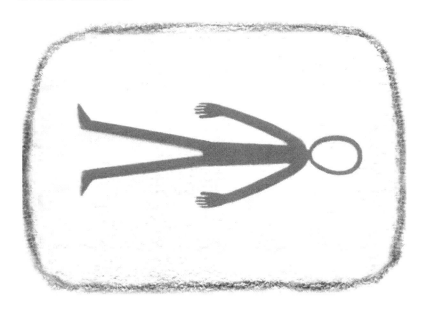

Movement:

You're lying flat on your back with your arms at your sides and your feet relaxed a comfortable distance apart. Breathe deeply—visualize oxygen being carried to every molecule and synapse of your body.

Here, in tranquil focus, enjoy affirmations of a love-sending and love-receiving day. Picture your intentions for the day, see them manifest according to your heart's desire. Move through your day in your mind's eye, meditatively, with equanimity, calmly sailing through even moments of challenge.

Picture yourself pausing to appreciate a flower, drinking in a work of art, stopping to listen to bird-song, and smiling warmly at others you encounter.

What a great day!

Or, if you're doing yoga at the end of the day, picture a deep and healing sleep, affirming that you will rest peacefully and heal fully.

Good Night! Sleep Tight!

After giving attention to your affirmations, release it all. Let it go. Become mindful of your breathing. Breathe deeply, inhaling and exhaling—stomach rising and falling. It's good to be mindful of total, deep, breathing.

Let everything go, relaxing. *Relax.*

There is nothing to worry about. There's nothing to do. Feel your mind relaxing. Your face relaxes. Your arms and your hands ... relax. Your chest and your abdomen ... relax. Your legs and your feet ... relax. *You completely ... relax....*

> You are the sky.
> Everything else is just weather.
> Pema Chodron

Let's Move!

After honoring your body with conscious relaxing (as distinguished from the unconscious relaxation of sleep, which may include grinding of teeth, clenched jaw, leg cramps, and general thrashing about, which is *not* entirely relaxed!) let's begin with some gentle, delicious movement.

Side Bend (reclined) – Urdhva Hastasana

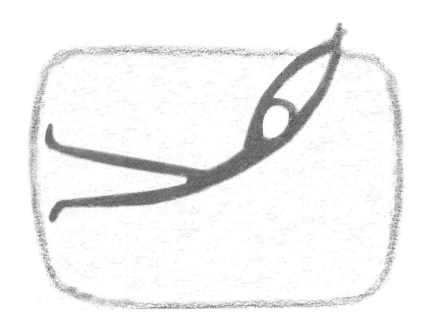

Movement:

From your *Shavasana*, move your legs a bit farther apart, then stretch your arms to full extension overhead. Hold on to your left wrist with your right hand, and bend to the right to the extent of your comfort, stretching your left side. Feel the stretch from your feet to your fingers.

Hold this position for several breaths. Breathe deeply, mindfully sensing your life-giving breath nurturing your ribs, your spinal cord, your brain, and your organs.

Take delight in the yummy feeling of your muscles stretching.

When you're ready, return to the center, then hold on to your right wrist with your left hand and bend to the left. Feel the stretch of your right side from your feet to your fingers. Sink into the lovely sensation and remain here for an equal amount of time as you stretched your left side.

Benefits:
Side bends activate your core muscles, expand your ribs, and deepen your breath, stimulating the flow of blood and energy through your organs, and improving circulation.

The movement increases the range of motion and elasticity of your spine, which in turn feeds your brain, stimulating the flow of cerebrospinal fluid.

Keeps you young and flexible!

There's a crack in everything....
That's how the light gets in.
Leonard Cohen

Bridge – Setu Bandha Sarvangasana

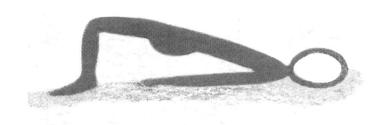

Movement:

Lie on your back with your feet hips-width apart and at a 90 degree angle under your knees, parallel to one another. Reach your arms along your sides and picture your collarbone wide. Relax into the moment, sensing where every part of your body is.

Rock a bit to the right, bringing your left shoulder blade in and down toward your left hip. Settle into the pose, then rock a bit to the left and bring your right shoulder blade in and down toward your right hip.

Now gently, but firmly, push down through your legs and into your feet, as if pushing the bed away from you. Curl your tailbone up as you rise, vertebra by vertebra, into your bridge. Breathe into this movement, and when your bridge reaches its pinnacle, slowly let it down, vertebra by vertebra, each in turn gently touching down.

Slowly and mindfully repeat the rising and lowering of your bridge, vertebra by vertebra, five to ten times.

Or, conversely, you may raise your bridge and hold it raised for a minute, or as long as it is comfortable.

Benefits:

Bridge pose has numerous benefits. It strengthens your legs, it opens your heart, it expands, relaxes, and strengthens your shoulders, and it nurtures the flexibility of your spine—all in an essentially relaxing position.

It's also a pose that gives you a good idea of your energy level. Some days you may have the energy to raise only a few vertebra into your bridge. Other days your bridge raises right to your shoulders without hesitation.

Your bridge is perfect, whatever its height. It's keeping your vertebra flexible, and opening your heart to healthy, enriching blood-flow as long as you mindfully inhale and exhale throughout the pose.

> Yoga is the journey of the self,
> Through the self,
> To the self.
> The Bhagavad Gita

Reclining Spinal Twist –
Jathara Parivartanasana

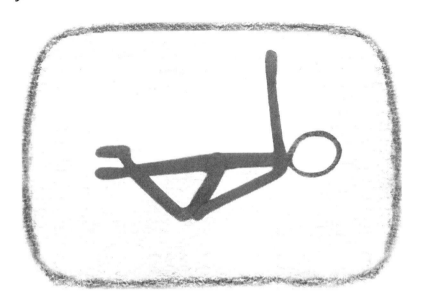

Movement:

Begin by hugging your knees to your chest, then slowly extend your left leg. Guide your bent right knee across your body with your left hand, gently relaxing your knee to the bed. You can put a pillow under your bent knee for support if it doesn't touch the bed.

Extend your right arm straight out from your body and turn your head to the right while keeping both shoulders touching the bed.

Inhale energy, exhale release, moving more deeply into the pose.

Feel your spine relaxing, let your shoulders melt in relaxation, feel your hip and your bent knee gently giving in to the reclining twist.

After one or two minutes relaxing into the twist, hug your knees, and repeat the sequence on the other side, slowly extending your right leg, then guiding your bent left knee across your body with your right hand, while extending your left arm.

Turn your head to the left, keeping your shoulders touching the bed.

Inhale energy, exhale release, moving more deeply into the pose.

Feel your spine relaxing, let your shoulders melt in relaxation, as your hip and bent knee gently give in to the reclining twist.

Hold the pose for a minute or two.

Benefits:
Twists help wring out toxins in your organs—and along with the toxins, the anxious and exhausted emotions that often accompany these toxins melt away.

Your *Reclining Spinal Twist* stimulates the flow of fresh blood to your digestive organs, while strengthening abdominal muscles and toning your waist. *Reclining*

Spinal Twist stretches your back muscles and glutes, while giving your back and hips a nice massage. Twists also hydrate, lengthen, relax and realign your spine.

A gentle spinal twist feels delicious first thing in the morning, or in the evening after a taxing day.

> Yoga revels in finding the movement in stillness
> And the stillness in movement.
>
> Blythe Ayne

Reclining Triangle – Utthita Trikonasana

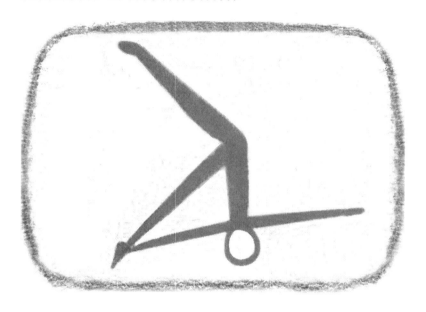

Movement:

Let's practice *Reclining Triangle,* a standing pose, in a reclined position. Move your feet wide apart, turning your left foot flat against the bed while keeping your right foot pointing up. With your legs straight, lift your knee caps, roll your left thigh out so your knee is in line with your big toe.

Draw your stomach in and stretch your arms out parallel to the top and the bottom of the bed, extending energetically right through to the ends of your fingertips.

Inhaling deeply, lengthen through both your right and your left ribs—don't "crunch" your left ribs—as you stretch toward your left foot. Place your hand wherever it rests comfortably, on your thigh, calf, or foot. Keep your neck in line with your spine and look up at your extended right hand, or down at your left foot if looking up strains your neck.

Relax into the pose, breathing deeply, extending through your fingertips and lengthening through the crown of your head. When you're ready to come out of the pose, return your arms parallel to the top and bottom of the bed, orient your feet in the opposite positions, and repeat the pose on the other side.

Either rest in the pose for a minute or two on each side, or move mindfully from one side to the other slowly, several times. Whichever you prefer, be sure to keep your legs engaged, lengthening through your ribs, your arms, and the crown of your head.

Benefits:
What's great about doing a standing pose in a reclined position is that if and when you take a standing pose to the floor, you've become familiar with how your body feels when in perfect alignment, as you're in perfect alignment with your back against the bed. The pose will be beautiful and beneficial, both reclining and standing.

Triangle pose stretches your thighs, hamstrings, calves, shoulders, chest, and spine, and is great for making your hips more flexible, while contributing to your sense of balance.

> If everyone did yoga
> We would have world peace.
> Rory Freedman

Staff Pose – Dandasana

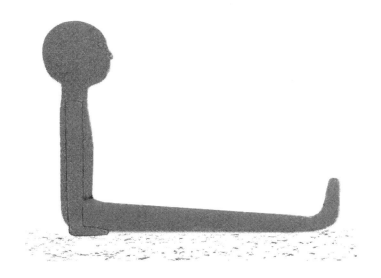

Movement

Staff pose is an active-without-movement pose. Sit with your legs together and outstretched. Keep your back perfectly straight with your hands facing forward next to your hips.

Flex your feet, pushing through your heels while actively pressing your sitting bones into the bed. Draw your abdomen in and up to help you sit straight.

Draw your shoulders down and toward each other, opening your chest. Be sure your shoulders are over your hips. Tuck your chin slightly, keeping your neck long and your ears in line with your shoulders.

Breathe deeply in this pose for several breaths with the abdominal muscles engaged, remaining active-yet-relaxed in the pose.

Benefits:
Staff Pose improves your core stability, strengthens your back muscles and your quads.

It improves your posture. It also sets you up for other upward facing poses.

You cannot always control
what goes on outside,
But you can control
what goes on inside.
Wayne Dyer

Seated Forward Bend – Paschimottanasana

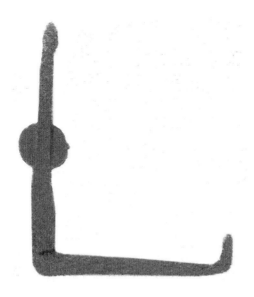

Movement:
Sit with your legs outstretched and your feet flexed. Inhale and lengthen your spine, then raise your arms straight overhead, alongside your ears.

Picture the front of your body open and long. Exhale and gently begin to fold forward, hinging from your hips, keeping the spine straight. Feel the movement in your chest, ribcage, and stomach as you move your forehead toward your legs.

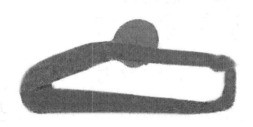

Reach your hands to the bottoms of your feet. If you can't reach your feet, bend your knees slightly until you can wrap your index finger and thumb around your big toes. Continue to gently extend your legs.

Inhale and exhale slowly and mindfully, concentrating on hinging at your hips. Keep your arms lifted, pull your shoulders away from your ears, while keeping your collar bones wide.

On the in-breath, lengthen the front of your torso. On the out-breath, fold deeper into the bend, hinging from the hips with a straight spine, keeping your neck in line with your spine.

Breathe into your *Seated Forward Bend* as long as it feels good.

Benefits:
The benefits of a relaxing-yet-mindful *Seated Forward Bend* are plentiful. It stretches the spine, shoulders and hamstrings.

It stimulates the organs and aids digestion.

It's therapeutic for insomnia, sinusitis, high blood pressure and depression.

Relax into a calm *Seated Forward Bend* any time stressors threaten to overwhelm you.

Yoga not only changes the way we see things ~
It transforms the person who sees.

Iyengar

Seated Twist – Half Lord of the Fishes
Ardha Matsyendrasana

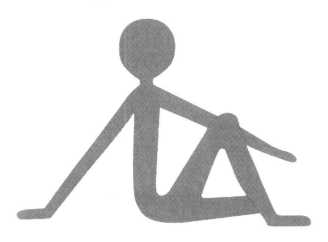

Movement:
Sit with your legs extended, spine straight. Bring your left foot on the outside of your right leg.

Then bend your right leg, bringing your right foot toward your left hip. If this is difficult in the beginning, you can leave your right leg straight.

Place your left hand behind your left hip. Inhale deeply and raise your right arm up, then hook it on the left side of your left knee. If this is difficult, simply hug your knee to your chest.

Picture your spine straight and your sitting bones even, your shoulders level and your collar bones wide.

Breathe deeply and mindfully. On your in-breath, lengthen your spine, on your out-breath, move gently further into the twist. Repeat this mindful lengthening and twisting for four to eight breaths. It's more important to lengthen your spine than to move into the twist.

On an out-breath, come out of the pose, extend both legs, then repeat on the other side.

Benefits:
Half Lord of the Fishes helps your spine maintain, and even *increase*, its range of motion.

It relives backache and sciatica.

It provides an excellent stretch for your hips, shoulders, and neck.

It squeezes toxins out of your organs and improves your digestion.

> The kindling of mindful movement
> Lights the fires of peace, wisdom & health.
> Blythe Ayne

Happy Baby – Ananda Balasana

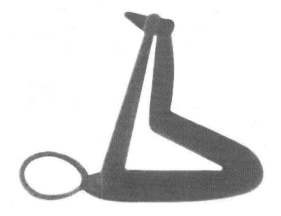

Movement:

Lie on your back and bring your knees over your chest, wider than your torso. Keep your ankles directly over your knees in a 90 degree angle. Flex your heels and grab the outside of your feet, pulling them, gently, toward you. Picture your thighs moving toward the bed, still wider than your torso.

Continue the resistance of pushing your feet into your hands, and your hands pulling down on your feet. Keep your spine lo-o-o-n-g by lengthening your tailbone, drawing your stomach in slightly, and keeping length in your neck.

Breathe deeply, and be a *Happy Baby!*—calm and grateful for your lovely toes in this relaxing, spine-healing pose. My teacher, Richard Matusow, said that he recently saw a baby doing this in a grocery store, guilelessly in *Happy Baby* pose. Be like that, simply *in the moment*.

Hold the pose until you're done with it. Then gently bring your feet back to the bed.

If you can't quite reach your feet yet, (you will eventually!), or if you have a knee or ankle injury, you can hold onto the back of your thighs.

If your neck feels sensitive or painful, support your head by placing a folded blanket under it.

Benefits:
Happy Baby stretches your spine, groin, and hips, while strengthening your arms.

It decompresses your sacroiliac joint, always a good thing, but particularly excellent for sciatica!

Happy Baby is calming, relieving fatigue and stress.

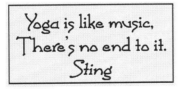

Yoga is like music,
There's no end to it.
Sting

Boat – Paripurna Navasana

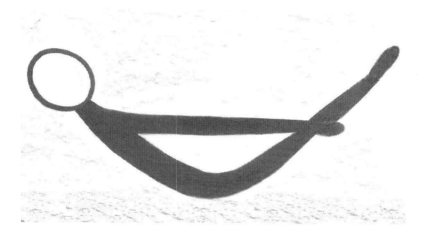

Movement:

Begin in a sitting position, with your knees bent, feet on the bed. Place your hands slightly behind your hips, hands facing forward.

Lengthen your spine, open your collar bones wide to open the chest while drawing in your abdominal muscles.

Lean back on your sitting bones and lift your feet, until your calves are parallel to the bed.

Keeping the spine straight and the chest open, extend your arms parallel to the bed. Picture your thigh bones, attached to your hip flexors, as anchors to the bottom of your spine, from which both your spine and your thighs raise in a strong "V." Breathe deeply into the pose.

At first you may not be able to raise your calves into a 45 degree angle. That will come with practice. What's important is to keep your spine and thighs in the 45 degree angle, while bending at the knees.

If you have lower back pain, move into boat pose gently. Though it will strengthen your lower back over time, do not engage in it to the point of pain.

Benefits:
Boat pose stimulates digestion and improves your core strength.

But most importantly, it strengthens your hip flexors that attach your inner thigh bones to the front of your spine.

Boat pose is also known for relieving stress.

> I close my eyes in order to see.
> Paul Gauguin

Fish – Matsyasana

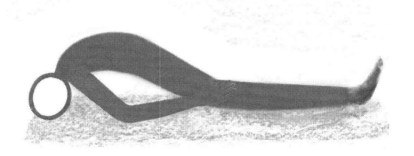

Movement:

Lying on your back, place your hands on the tops of your thighs. You may extend your toes or flex them, but either way, keep your feet and your toes engaged.

Inhale deeply while pressing your elbows into the bed. Lifting your chest, pull your shoulders together. Continue raising your chest until the top of your head rests on the bed. *The weight is in your elbows, not the top of your head!*

Relax into this pose for several deep breaths.

To come out of *Fish* pose, press with your elbows while gently lifting and relaxing your head on the bed.

If this pose is a challenge, place a pillow or folded blanket underneath your shoulders, and release your head over the edge of the pillow or blanket.

Benefits:

Fish pose stretches the intercostal muscles between the ribs, opens the chest, and opens and stimulates the throat.

It opens your breathing and is energizing. It has an amazing ability to relieve irritation and that "grindy" feeling one gets from over-stimulation, frustration, and, simply, those "bad traffic" days.

> Yoga teaches you how to listen to your body.
>
> Mariel Hemingway

Reclining Butterfly –
Supta Baddha Konasana

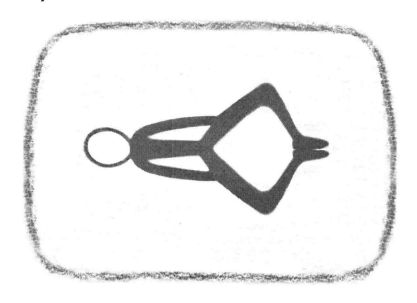

Movement:

In a seated position, bring the soles of your feet together, with your legs in a diamond shape. Lie back on the bed, placing your hands on your abdomen, thighs, or out to your sides on the bed.

Relax into your *Reclined Butterfly*. You can use pillows under your knees for support if your inner thighs are uncomfortable. Breathe deeply while your spine and knees relax.

If your lower back is arching, prop up on your elbows to keep your spine long and flat on the bed.

Eventually you will be able to stay in *Reclined Butterfly*, spine long, knees relaxed, in a gentle pose for as long as it feels restorative.

Benefits:
Reclined Butterfly is great for relaxing, as well as having several benefits. It increases the mobility in your hips.

It stimulates the bladder and kidney meridians.

It reduces stress, calms your mind, and alleviates insomnia.

In yoga, where your body has the greatest resistance
Is where there'll be the greatest breakthrough.
So it is in life.

Blythe Ayne

Easy Pose – Sukhasana

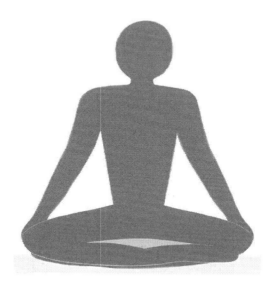

Movement:

Sit on a firm folded blanket so that your hips are in line with, or a bit above your knees, and cross your shins so that they are parallel to the end of the bed, with each foot underneath the opposite knee. You may not initially be able to bring each foot under the opposite knee. Come as close as you can—it *will* get easier as you practice. You can add a blanket or pillow to the one you're sitting on to raise your hips yet higher, which may be helpful.

Straighten and lengthen your spine, while pushing your sitting bones into the folded blanket, creating length through your spine to the crown of your head.

Firm your shoulder blades and place your hands in your lap or on your knees, palms down for a calming effect, or up for energizing.

Relax in this position for as long as it feels beneficial. For variety in the pose, cross your legs the opposite way, which will feel awkward, but is very good for both your brain and your flexibility.

Benefits:
Easy Pose or *Happy Sitting Pose* as it's also called, strengthens your back, opens your hips, calms your mind, and is good for preparing you to do breathing exercises or to meditate.

> The soul is here for its own joy.
> Rumi

Cow Face – Gomukhasana

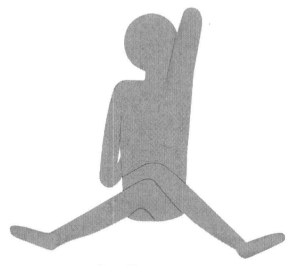

Cow Face - Front

Movement:

Start in *Staff Pose,* with your legs straight out in front of you and your spine straight. Inhaling deeply, cross your right knee over your left knee, bringing your right foot to the outside of your left hip. Then bend your left knee, bringing your left foot to the outside of your right hip. The goal is to have your knees stacked one over the other in alignment, although initially they may not yet be willing to do that.

Make sure both of your sitting bones are grounded evenly on the bed, with your heels each an equal distance from your hips. It's important that you sit squarely, which is the challenge in *Cow Face* as the top knee will raise that hip if you don't consciously ground it.

If you can't get both hips to sit evenly, sit on a pillow or folded blanket, which will raise your hips and make it easier to keep them in line. As you continue to practice *Cow Face*, your heels will come closer to your hips.

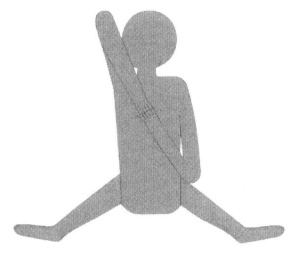

Cow Face - Back

Next, inhale and stretch your arms out to the sides, palms facing forward. Exhaling, turn your right thumb facing down and bring your right arm behind your back, walking it up between your shoulder blades, palm facing out.

Then inhale and stretch your left arm up, palm facing forward. Exhale, bend your elbow, and reach down between your shoulder blades. The goal is to hook your right fingers with your left fingers—*eventually!*

You can use a stretch band or a scarf in your upper hand that your lower hand grasps, working to bring your two hands closer together. At the same time, keep your elbow close to your torso.

Firm your shoulders against your back to open your chest and heart, keeping your spine straight from the crown of your head to your sitting bones. Stay in the pose for a few deep, relaxing breaths.

Then release your arms, straighten your legs, and repeat the same movements on the other side. Don't be surprised if you discover *Cow Face* is easier to accomplish on one side than the other. This is so with most yoga poses, but *Cow Face* tends to highlight that difference. It's good to know your stronger side and your weaker side, so you can nurture each accordingly.

Over time, as you become more flexible in the pose, you can begin to fold forward, keeping the spine straight and the weight in your sitting bones. This is an advanced version of the pose, *so don't rush it!* Be with your *Cow Face*, right where it is, in the moment.

Benefits:
Cow Face stretches your ankles, thighs and hips. It works your upper back and chest muscles, as well as your triceps and rotator cuff. It opens both your chest and your thoracic spine, while strengthening the spine, the abdominals, and stimulating the kidneys.
Cow Face helps you become relaxed, relieving tension throughout the body.

> To perform every action artfully
> Is yoga.
> Swami Kripalu

Seated Side Angle Bend –
Parsva Upavistha Konasana

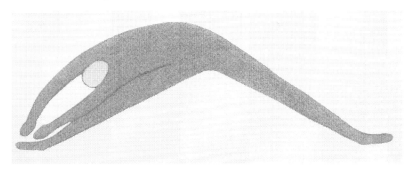

Movement:

From *Staff Pose*, sitting with your spine long, and your legs straight out in front, move your legs into as wide an angle as you comfortably can, while keeping the integrity of your straight spine. If you feel your lower back bowing out, sit on a folded blanket.

Flex your feet, keeping your knees and toes pointed up. Press your legs and sitting bones down while lengthening through your spine, tilting your pubic bone up and back to assist in keeping the spine straight.

Twist from your waist to face your right leg. As you exhale, walk your hand toward your right foot, while reaching your forehead toward your knee. The goal is to hold onto your right foot, but if you're not there yet, hold onto your shin or ankle. When you reach your pose, relax your elbows, shoulders, and neck.

If you have reached your foot, you can deepen the pose by pressing out through your heel and pulling your toes toward you. Hold for several breaths, relaxing into the pose.

Release the pose by slowly walking your hands back to your waist and gently rolling up your spine, returning to your seated staff pose. Then repeat the movements on your left side.

Benefits:
Seated Side Angle Bend opens and stretches your hips and the backs of your legs, while strengthening your spine.

It stimulates the abdominal organs and provides deep relaxation.

The essence of yoga
Is the union between individual consciousness
And divine consciousness.
Raphael

Seated Wide-Angle Forward Bend – Upavistha Konasana

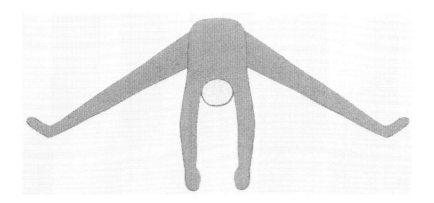

Movement:

Wide-Angle Seated Forward Fold begins the same as *Seated Side Angle Bend*. From *Staff Pose*, sitting with your spine long, and your legs straight out in front, move your legs into as wide an angle as you comfortably can, while keeping the integrity of your straight spine. If you feel your lower back bowing out, sit on a folded blanket.

Flex your feet, keeping your knees and toes pointed up. Press your legs and sitting bones down while lengthening through your spine, tilting your pubic bone up and back to assist in keeping the spine straight. Begin to bend from your hips, not your back, and place your hands in front of you on the bed. Slowly exhale, pushing your hands forward.

Keep the front of your body long and straight as you come forward, lengthening from pubic bone to breast bone. When you feel your back begin to arch, pause, breathing deeply. On an exhalation, move deeper into the pose if you can. When you reach your limit of stretching your hands forward while keeping your back straight, you will feel the stretch along the back of your legs.

Stay in this pose for several breaths, feeling the energy of the stretch in your legs. Then return to your seated position, coming up with a straight back, while pressing your sitting bones down.

Benefits:
Wide-Angle Seated Forward Bend opens and stretches the back of your body, your hips, and the inside of your legs, while strengthening your spine.

It stimulates the abdominal organs and provides deep relaxation.

> Surrender to the moment
> It will tell you where to move
> To make the change you desire.
> Blythe Ayne

Excellent Work!

You've made your way through the upward and seated poses, take a well-earned break with your legs up the wall, before moving on the downward facing and reclining warrior poses.

Legs Up the Wall – Viparita Karani

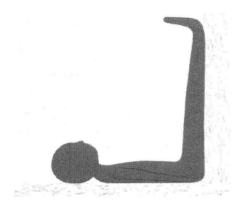

Movement:

Begin by moving your left side up against the wall, or head-board. Get as close to the wall as you can. Then lift your legs and gently rotate to the left, resting your legs on the wall. Using your hands to help support you, rock from side to side toward the wall, until the full extension of your legs is against the wall.

Relax your arms at your sides, palms facing up. Relax your legs, your feet, your calves, your thighs, relax your abdomen, your chest, your head, your arms and hands— just r-e-l-a-x. Breathe deeply, and remain in the pose for several minutes, enjoying the relaxation and rejuvenation.

To come out of the pose, slide your legs down to your right, and gently use your hands to turn around and return to a seated position.

Alternatively, you can do legs up, without the wall. Although it doesn't provide the same total relaxation, it does offer the advantages of inversions—see *Inversions*, below.

Benefits:

Although a completely relaxed position, *Legs Up the Wall* has numerous benefits for mind, body, and spirit. Ancient texts say this pose will destroy old age. It stretches the back of your legs, and relieves cramps in legs and feet, while reducing swollen ankles and calves. It stretches your torso and the back of your neck.

Legs Up the Wall relieves:
Anxiety, headaches, migraine, backaches, insomnia, mild depression, muscle fatigue, arthritis, both high and low blood pressure, varicose veins, and cramps.

And *Legs Up the Wall* strengthens your immune system, balances your hormonal system, calms your nervous system, stabilizes your digestive and elimination systems, and regulates your respiratory system.

Inversions:

Inversions lower high blood pressure and improve blood circulation, which provides more oxygen and blood to the brain, augmenting memory, concentration, and mental processing. Just three to five minutes of inversion allows the tired blood of your lower limbs to flow rapidly back to the heart, where it refreshes.

In an inversion, tissue fluids can flow more efficiently into the veins and lymph system of your lower limbs and abdominal and pelvic organs, providing a healthy exchange of nutrients and wastes between cells and capillaries.

> Yoga is a dance between
> Control and surrender.
> Joel Kramer

Tabletop – Bharmanasana

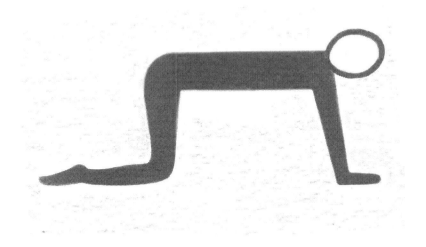

Movement:

From a hands and knees position, have your knees hips distance apart and your feet directly in line with your knees. Your hands are shoulder width apart, with fingers pointing forward, pressing down and actively engaged.

Look down between your palms, picturing your spine in a straight line. Pull your shoulders back and away from your ears. Energetically pull your tailbone toward the wall behind you, while pressing the crown of your head toward the front wall.

While in stillness, continue to engage your spine.

Benefits:

Tabletop is great for realigning and lengthening your spine. It's also a key posture for transitioning to several other postures.

> The future depends
> On what we do in the present.
> Mahatma Gandhi

Cat – Marjariasana

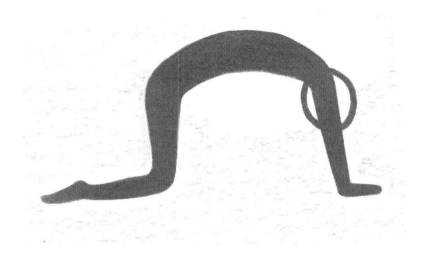

Movement:

From tabletop on your hands and knees, inhale deeply, and as you exhale, round your spine upward, lifting through your waist and ribs.

Pull in your abdominal muscles while tucking your tailbone. Gently release the crown of your head toward the bed, while continuing to press firmly through your palms and fingers. Drop your shoulders away from your ears.

Breathe into your *Cat* pose as long as it feels luscious.

Benefits:
Cat pose is a great stretch for your back and neck. While gently massaging the spine, it also increases circulation of spinal fluid and mobility.

It's great for your wrists, stimulating their blood circulation. This is especially fantastic after a long stint at the computer.

Cat pose helps relieve stress.

> Your yoga is where you are.
> Not where you were or will be.
> Blythe Ayne

Cow – Bitilasana

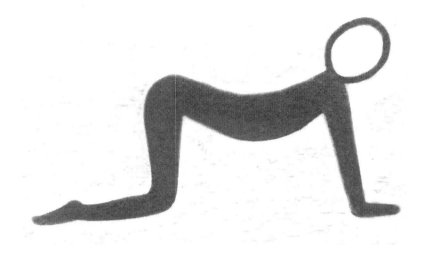

Movement:

Return to your *Tabletop* position, knees under hips and wrists under shoulders.

Inhale lifting your sitting bones upwards, while opening your chest and allowing your abdominals and belly to sink toward the bed. Lift your head and look forward or up, but be careful not to crunch the back of your neck when you look up. Drop your shoulders away from your ears.

Enjoy the release in *Cow* for several breaths, then return to *Tabletop*.

Benefits:

Cow stretches your middle to low back, your hips, your neck, and the front of your torso.

It massages your spine and your internal organs, while stimulating your kidneys and adrenal glands.

Cat-Cow Flow
Movement:

A *Cat-Cow* flow is a delicious warm-up before your regular yoga practice. Move from *Cat* into *Cow*, and from *Cow* back to *Cat* at a pace that feels just right for the moment—it's an excellent flow to limber up your spine before yoga, or anytime!

> Do not feel lonely.
> The entire universe is inside you.
> Rumi

Dolphin –
Ardha Pincha Mayurasnana

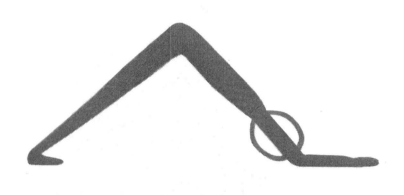

Movement:

From your *Tabletop*, all fours position, making sure your knees are directly below your hips, place your forearms on the bed, with your shoulders directly above your elbows. Open your shoulders wide, and press the length of your forearms into the bed.

Inhale deeply. On your exhale, curl your toes under and lift your knees. Keep your knees slightly bent, with more attention given to keeping your spine long and straight.

Gradually straighten your legs and reach your heels toward the bed. Continue to picture your spine straight, while drawing the muscles of your legs in and up.

Extend your hips upward, and pull your shoulder blades down, maintaining the width between them. Keep your neck relaxed, aligned with your spine, and align your head with your arms.

Hold this position for several deep breaths, visualizing your spine straight, with each vertebra and disk being nurtured by the reverse flow of blood and spinal fluid in the space between each of them.

Benefits:
This is an excellent alternate pose for *Downward Dog*, while easier to accomplish on a bed.

Dolphin strengthens and stretches your shoulders, arms, and legs, and is great for the arches of your feet. It improves digestion and calms the mind, while helping to relieve stress and depression.

> Yoga is when every cell of the body sings the song of the soul.
>
> Iyengar

Locust – Salabasana

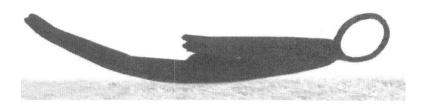

Movement:

Lie on your stomach with your arms stretched out along your sides, palms down, head relaxed, facing down.

Lengthen your lower back and pull your navel in toward your spine. Exhaling, engage your leg muscles.

Inhaling, lift your head, arms, upper chest, and legs. Keep your chin slightly tucked to avoid crunching the back of your neck. Push through the balls of your feet and firm your shoulders, opening your heart. Pretend someone is holding onto your hands, pulling back and lifting you further up.

Hold this pose for three to five calm, deep, breaths, then exhale, relaxing down onto the bed. Repeat locust pose one or two more times, then completely relax, making a pillow of your forearms.

When first practicing locust, it may be difficult to lift your legs. Do the pose a couple of times, only lifting your arms, while picturing lifting your legs, then lift your legs on the third try. Or lift one leg for three to five breaths, lower it, then lift the other leg for three to five breaths.

Benefits:
Locust is a great pose to strengthen your back and leg muscles.

It also stimulates your abdominal organs, while giving the front of your body a good stretch.

> Find the place inside yourself
> Where nothing is impossible.
> Deepak Chopra

Bow – Dhanurasana

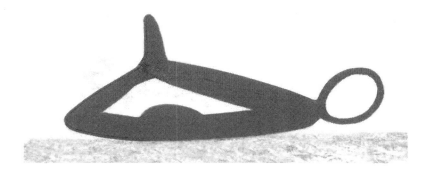

Movement:

Lie on your stomach with your arms along your sides, palms up.

Exhale, bending your knees as much as you can, and grab your ankles with your hands. Keep your knees together or no more than hips-width apart.

Pull your navel toward your spine, and push your ankles into your hands, lifting your thighs, chest, and head, chin slightly tucked, keeping the back of your neck long. Press your shoulder blades into your back to open your heart.

Breathe deeply into your back for several breaths before releasing gently and with control.

Make a pillow with your forearms and relax fully, inhaling and exhaling deeply.

If reaching both of your ankles is difficult, roll gently to your left and grab your right ankle, pressing your ankle into your hand, breathing deeply for a few breaths.

Then release and roll gently to the right, grabbing your left ankle. Press it into your hand, breathing deeply an equal number of breaths as on the left.

Benefits:
Bow pose strengthens your back, opens your chest, and stretches the front of your body.

It energizes your whole body, stimulates your organs, and eases anxiety.

> Yoga is the perfect opportunity
> To be curious about who you are.
> Jason Crandell

Cobra – Bhujangasana

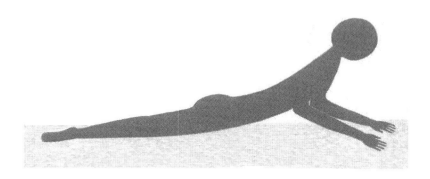

Movement:

Lie on your stomach, toes pointing back, elbows close to your ribs, and your hands under your shoulders, forehead on the bed. Engage your legs and pull your stomach in.

Inhale and lift your torso, firming your shoulder blades into your upper back, pulling them toward your spine. Then lift your head and open your chest, but have no weight on your hands. Extend this back bend out through your toes.

Ease down on an exhale. Repeat this movement again. Then, the next time you rise up, use your hands to come up higher. Lift your chest first, then your head, in an upward rolling motion.

Keep your shoulders drawn down away from your ears. Firm your tailbone and come up as far as it feels good, keeping the legs engaged all the way through your toes.

Bring your ribs forward, draw your upper arms back and keep your elbows touching your ribs. Lengthen your neck and extend the backbend through your entire spine.

Hold the pose for several breaths, and then relax, making a pillow of your forearms.

Benefits:
Cobra strengthens your arms, shoulders, upper back and legs, while giving the front of your body a good stretch.

It's an energizing pose, and relieves mild depression.

> Yoga is the process by which
> Transformation is achieved.
> Srivatsa Ramaswami

Pigeon –
Utthita Eka Pada Kapotasana

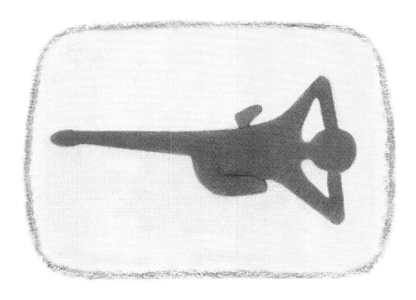

Movement:

From *Tabletop* on all fours, hands under shoulders and knees under hips, bring your right knee forward and place it behind your right wrist, with your ankle in front of your left hip. Try to get your shin in a straight line behind your two hands, though this may be difficult at first.

Slide your left leg straight behind you, making sure that it's not drawing out to the side. Straighten your left knee and point your toes. Keep the right foot flexed.

Gently lower your torso over your bent leg. Keep your hips level with one another—the tendency is for the crossed leg to lower that hip. Place a pillow or folded blanket under your right hip if it is difficult to get your hips to stay level.

Be mindful of your bent knee. If this pose troubles your knees, you can do it lying on your back, extending your left leg on the bed and holding your right bent leg across your torso with your hands.

Breathing deeply, stay in *Pigeon* for several breaths, continuing to release the tension in the right hip.

To come out of the pose, push yourself up with your hands and return to all fours. Then repeat the movement on the other side.

Benefits:
Pigeon pose opens your hips, using core strength to keep your hips level, while stretching your thighs, psoas and groin. Fully relaxing into *Pigeon* is a wonderfully calming pose.

> Live life
> As if everything is set up in your favor.
> Rumi

Child's Pose – Balasana

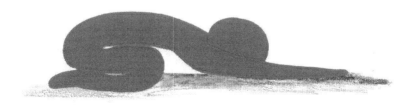

Movement:

Kneel on the bed with your knees in alignment with your hips, or wider, and your big toes touching. Exhaling, relax your stomach between your thighs, while pulling back onto your heels, or as close to them as possible.

Extend your arms in front as far as they will reach. To keep the pose active, raise your elbows off the bed. To fully relax in the pose, let your elbows relax.

Conversely, you may reach your arms back along your torso, palms up, relaxing your shoulders toward the bed.

Rest your forehead on the bed. If your head does not easily rest on the bed, use pillows to raise your head until you can rest comfortably. Stay in this resting pose for as long as it feels good. Return to *Child's Pose* any time during your yoga practice you need a few moments to relax and recharge.

Benefits:

Along with being an excellent few moments of relaxation, *Child's Pose* gently stretches your shoulders, lower back, hips, thighs, ankles and knees.

It helps to relieve fatigue, increases blood circulation to your head, and calms your mind and body.

Sometimes not getting what you want
Is a wonderful stroke of luck.
Dalai Lama

Warrior I Pose – Verabhadrasana I

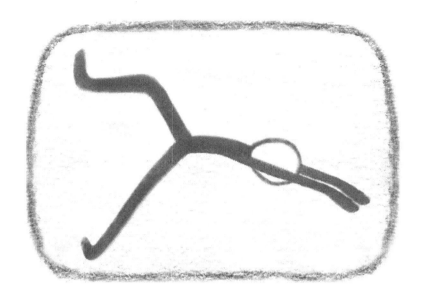

Movement:

Let's take the *Warrior Poses* to the bed! As previously mentioned, the advantage of practicing standing poses while lying down is that, although they're not the same as when weight bearing, you'll get the *feel* of your body in proper alignment. This can be a significant advantage when you take these poses to the floor.

Move down on the bed far enough to be able to raise your arms overhead. Lying on your right side, stretch your legs into a wide "V." Place a folded blanket under your left foot, so that it's a bit higher than your right foot, and turn your left foot so your toes point to the ceiling. Your right foot is lying flat on the bed so that your feet are perpendicular to one another. Bend your right knee to a 90 degree angle.

Roll your right hip back, and your left hip forward so they are in line with one another, while keeping your torso in a straight line over your hips. Engage your leg muscles.

Inhale and lift your arms overhead, pulling your shoulders down away from your ears. Elongate your spine, open your collarbones, and lift your breastbone. Firm your triceps to raise your arms further.

Hold the pose for ten or fifteen slow breaths, or longer if it feels beneficial, then relax onto your back, bringing your feet together and your arms to your sides. Repeat the movements on your left side.

Benefits:
Warrior I opens your hip joints and helps to alleviate painful conditions involving the sacrum. It improves posture and stretches your ankles, calves and thighs.

It improves the mobility in your shoulders, while opening your chest and lungs.

Warrior poses augment your mind-body connection, opening the heart to stimulate emotional strength.

The warrior poses also support the parasympathetic nervous system, which in turn sustains equanimity.

The power of imagination
Makes you infinite.
John Muir

Humble Warrior – Baddha Verabhadrasana

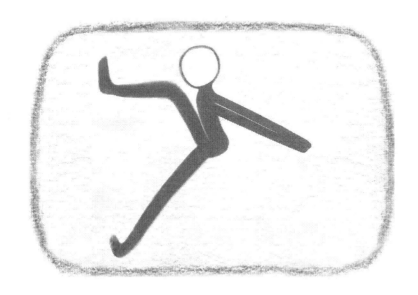

Movement:

Humble Warrior takes its stance from *Warrior I*. Lying on your right side, stretch your legs into a wide "V." Place a folded blanket under your left foot, so that it's a bit higher than your right foot, and turn your left foot so your toes point to the ceiling. Your right foot is lying flat on the bed and your feet are perpendicular to one another. Bend your right knee to a 90 degree angle.

Roll your right hip back, and your left hip forward so they are in line with one another, while keeping your torso squarely over your hips. Engage your leg muscles.

Reaching your arms behind your back, bring your torso toward your front bent knee. Bring your chest into contact with your thigh if possible, and raise your clasped hands further behind your back. Keep your legs, arms, and torso engaged while you remain in this pose.

Humble Warrior Variation:

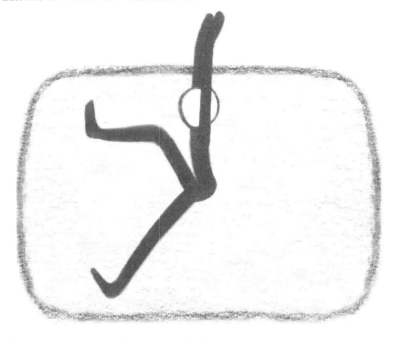

If your arms reaching up behind you is too uncomfortable, reach your arms forward instead, while extending your torso toward your knee. Keep your legs, arms, and torso engaged in this pose.

Benefits:

Humble Warrior opens your lungs and chest and stretches your arms, legs, back and neck. It is a deep hip opener, and a shoulder opener when your hands are clasped behind your back.

It stimulates the nervous system and the abdominal organs. It stimulates feelings of quiet strength and inspires equanimity and acceptance.

No yoga
No peace.
Know yoga
Know peace.
R. C. Seth

Warrior II Pose – Verabhadrasana II

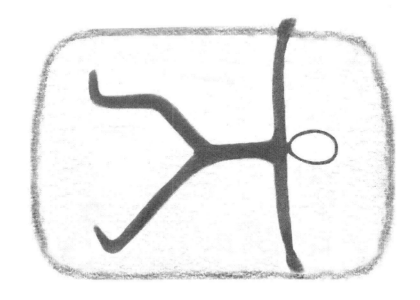

Movement:

Lying flat on your back, move your legs apart to a wide-legged stance, and, on an inhale, raise your arms to shoulder level, keeping your shoulders down and your neck long. Exhale and bend your right knee until it is in line with your ankle.

Engage your hips and elongate through the length of your spine. Draw your abdomen in and up while keeping your diaphragm soft. Extend from your collarbones out through the tips of your fingers. Draw your tailbone toward your feet to lengthen your lower back. Be sure that your shoulders are in line with your hips.

Fix your gaze beyond your right fingertips, imagining a bright and calm future.

Remain in this meditative pose for as long as it feels energizing. Relax from the pose by returning your arms to your sides and your legs extended straight, then repeat the sequence on the other side.

Benefits:
Warrior II opens your hips and stretches your thighs, chest, lungs, and shoulders, and increases stamina.

Warrior II opens your heart to wisdom, and steadies your intention, bringing a centered power to your daily life.

Listen to the quiet.

Blythe Ayne

Reverse Warrior Pose – Viparita Verabhadrasana

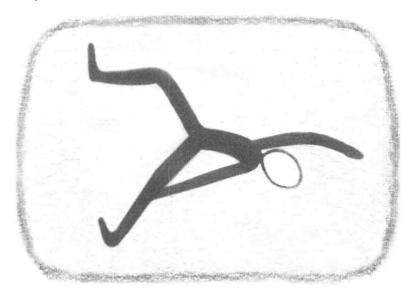

Movement:

Reverse Warrior starts in a *Warrior II* stance. Lying flat on your back, move your legs apart to a wide-legged stance, and, on an inhale, raise your arms to shoulder level, keeping your shoulders down and your neck long. Exhale and bend your right knee until it is in line with your ankle.

Engage your hips and elongate through the length of your spine. Draw your abdomen in and up, while keeping your diaphragm soft. Extend from your collarbones out through the tips of your fingers. Draw your tailbone toward your feet to lengthen your lower back. Be sure that your shoulders are in line with your hips.

Turn the palm of your right hand up. Inhaling, extend your arm above your head, while sliding your left arm down your left leg. Firm your shoulder blades, lift your chest and come into a gentle backbend. Raise your head and gaze at your right hand breathing deeply for several breaths.

Gently return to *Warrior II,* then repeat the movements on your left side.

Benefits:
Reverse Warrior opens your chest, side body, hips, groin and legs.

It releases tension in the intercostal muscles around your ribs and encourages deeper breathing. It's relaxing while at the same time, energizing.

Namaste ~
The Light in me
Recognizes and honors
The Light in you.

Congratulations!

You've worked your way through **Bed Yoga**—well done! It's time to return to your well-earned *Shavasana*, complete relaxation, while your body, mind, and spirit integrate all the wonderful work you've done.

Shavasana—total relaxation while conscious—is the whole point of yoga, to mindfully, yet in a relaxed state, let every cell of your body rejuvenate.

Shavasana

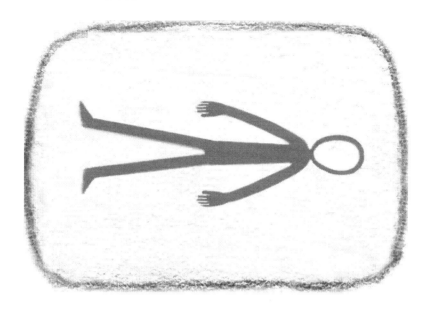

Movement:

You're lying flat on your back with your arms at your sides and your feet relaxed a comfortable distance apart. Breathe deeply—visualize oxygen being carried to every nook and cranny of your body.

Here, in tranquil focus, enjoy affirmations of a love-sending and love-receiving day. Picture your intentions for the day, see them manifest according to your heart's desire. Move through your day in your mind's eye, meditatively, with equanimity, sailing through even moments of challenge.

Picture yourself pausing to appreciate a flower, drinking in a work of art, stopping to listen to bird-song, and smiling warmly at others you encounter.

What a great day!

Or, if you're doing yoga at the end of the day, picture a deep and healing sleep, affirming that you will rest peacefully and heal fully.

Good Night! Sleep Tight!

After giving attention to your affirmations, release it all. Let it go. Become mindful of your breathing. Breathe deeply, inhaling and exhaling—stomach rising and falling. It's good to be mindful of total, deep, breathing.

Let everything go, relaxing. *Relax.*

There is nothing to worry about. There's nothing to do. Feel your mind relaxing. Your face relaxes. Your arms and your hands ... relax. Your chest and your abdomen ... relax. Your legs and your feet ... relax. *You completely ... relax....*

> You are the sky.
> Everything else is just weather.
> Pema Chodron

Yoga Flow

Breathing Exercises

Forms of Yoga

Your Yoga Routines

Yoga Flow

Flow happens when your strength, energy, thoughts, and feelings are integrated, moving in the same direction, with the same *intention*, and a focused *attention*, on the same path.

It's a sense of *hooking up*—whether it's your body, your mind, your heart's desires, your day, your entire life, or all of the foregoing. The result of flow is a feeling of being in the right place, doing the right thing, at the right time.

Flow in yoga is a series of physical movements that encourage the practice of flow in your thoughts (mind) and feelings (heart), providing the numerous benefits of stretching, integration, and purpose.

Flow in mind and body reinforces equanimity and a happy, productive, calm, meditative, and peaceful life.

In yoga
You can be a tree.
Blythe Ayne

Forms of Yoga

There are many forms of yoga, with each their own emphasis. But there are two processes to keep in mind, no matter what form you engage in:

Stay focused on your breath—inhale and exhale through your nose to maintain your body warmth and energy.

Visualize your spine—picture a comfortable space between each vertebra and disk. See, in your mind's eye, each vertebra, each disk, flexible in movement and in stillness, in perfect alignment, balanced and whole.

Many of us have vertebra or disks that are *not* in perfect alignment, that are *not* perfectly whole, but keeping that image in your mind's eye—which is a powerful source of healing, behind *your third eye!*—can contribute to your body's ability to maintain, and to heal.

Following is a short list of the more common forms of yoga:

Hatha Yoga is best for the beginner as it uses a variety of the common poses. It's a classic approach to yoga's poses and breathing exercises.

Iyengar Yoga was founded by B. K. S. Iyengar. It focuses on precise movements, and the details of alignment. Poses are generally held for a long period, while continuing to adjust the fine details of the pose.

Ashtanga Yoga the "Eight Limb path," is a physically demanding sequence of postures, generally more appropriate for the experienced yogi.

Vinyasa Yoga comes from *Ashtanga* as a flowing link of movements, united to the breath. It's not uncommon for a *Vinyasa* flow to be included in *Hatha* Yoga.

Restorative Yoga This book, *Bed Yoga*, takes a restorative approach. *Restorative Yoga* relaxes you, and, as its name implies, it restores you, body and mind and spirit. In this relaxation and restoration, there is also rejuvenation.

No matter what time of day you engage in *Restorative Yoga*, you'll reap the benefit of the three *R's*:
Relaxation
Restoration
Rejuvenation

> Light tomorrow with today.
> Elizabeth Barrett Browning

Pranayama – Yoga Breathing

What if you had to consciously breathe, telling your body to do everything it requires to take a breath?

Your body is *such a miracle!* Breathing, breathing, breathing, without having to give it a moment's thought. So those times when you *do* consciously think about your breath, send gratitude to your body for breathing without being instructed.

Breathing is the most natural thing our bodies do, generously providing the fuel of life-sustaining oxygen. Breathing relieves tension and stress, calms the nervous system, diminishes fatigue, stress, and high blood pressure with every inhale. It carts off carbon dioxide and toxins with every exhale. All accomplished automatically.

However, central to yoga practice is *conscious attention to your breath*, altering it so that it activates your parasympathetic nervous system, the "rest and digest" system—the opposite of "fight or flight," where our harried lives hurl us far too often.

"Prana" is your *Life Force,* regulated by your breath. When we breathe consciously, it takes us into a grounded and meditative state. There are a number of breathing exercises in yoga, let's consider three of the most common ones: *Ujjayi, Nadi Shodhana,* and *Kapalabhati.*

Ujjayi Breath

"Ujjayi" is Sanskrit for "victorious" or "to gain mastery." *Ujjayi* breath sounds like the ocean when it "inhales" coming into shore, and then "exhales," going back out to sea. In fact, this image of the ocean tide coming and going with your breath can help you stay focused on your breathing during your yoga practice.

How to Create Ujjayi Breath
You develop your *Ujjayi* breath by constricting the back of your throat, like when you're about to whisper. *Which you are!* Except you're not going to whisper words, you're going to whisper your breath as you breathe your *Ujjayi* breath through your nose.

Breathe in, slowly and deeply, hear the ocean coming in to the shore. There's a pause at the top of your breath, and then, slowly release your breath as the wave leaves the shore, returning out to the ocean. Then another pause at the bottom of your breath. Just like the tide, your breath returns again as it flows in and out through your nose.

So relaxing and calming....

Ujjayi Breath with Your Yoga Movements
Here are a few of the reasons why it's good to use *Ujjayi* breath with your yoga movements:

Ujjayi breathing improves concentration during your practice. When you are absorbed in producing your ocean breath, you can remain in poses for longer periods.

Ujjayi breathing releases tension both physically and mentally.

Ujjayi breathing is meditative and deepens the mind-body-spirit connection that is central to yoga. It assists in grounding you and nurtures your self-awareness.

Ujjayi breathing promotes regulated heat for your body. The friction of the air as it passes through your lungs and throat generates internal body heat. This warmed air massages your internal organs, making stretching even more enjoyable, and the positions more readily achieved.

This generated internal heat helps your organs clear out toxins.

Ujjayi Breath and Your Health
You may also discover that *Ujjayi* breath diminishes headaches, relieves sinus pressure and decreases phlegm, all while providing strength for your nervous and digestive systems.

The full, deep, breath of *Ujjayi* breathing helps with the challenges of a yoga practice. As your breathing habit develops, you may discover that it helps with challenges elsewhere in your life as well.

The ancient yogis knew that there's an intimate connection between *breath* and *mind*. Your breath is a teacher. As you learn to pay attention to it, you'll learn much about yourself, encouraging equanimity and strength through all of life's passages.

Nadi Shodhana – Alternate Nostril Breath

Nadi Shodhana comes from two Sanskrit words: *Nadi* = "flow" or "channel," and *Shodhana* = "purification." This breath exercise is focused on clearing the subtle channels of your body, mind, and spirit, while balancing your masculine and feminine energies.

How to Create Nadi Shodhana Breath

Sitting comfortably, keep your back, head, and neck in a straight line. Calmly take three or four deep breaths to become centered. Leave your left hand on your knee. Form the *Vishnu mudra* with your right hand by folding the index and middle fingers to your palm. Alternately, you may place your index and middle fingers between your eyebrows.

Inhale deeply, then with your right thumb, close off your right nostril. Exhale through your left nostril, picturing your breath traveling down the left side of your head, throat, down the left side of your spine through your organs, and down to your pelvic floor. Pause for a moment. Then inhale through your left nostril, picturing your breath traveling up from your pelvic floor up your left side, through all your organs, along the left side of your spine, and up into your throat and head. Pause.

Closing off your left nostril with your ring and pinky fingers, release your right nostril, and exhale, picturing your breath traveling down the right side of your head, throat, down the right side of your spine through your organs, and down to your pelvic floor. Pause. Then inhale through your right nostril, picturing your breath traveling up from your pelvic floor up your right side, through all your organs, along the right side of your spine, and up into your throat and head.

Continue this cycle for 20 or 30 breaths, then complete with an exhalation through your left nostril, and relax your right hand in your lap or on your knee and breathe deeply.

A variation is to count on the inhalation up to a comfortable number, for example six, hold the breath for a count of two, then exhale for a count of six and hold at the bottom of your breath for a count of two. An alternate discipline for this method is to increase the count on the exhalation and inhalation.

Nadi Shodhana Breath and Your Health

Nadi Shodhana has many benefits. It removes toxins while infusing your body with oxygen. It reduces stress and anxiety. It clears your respiratory channels, and helps to alleviate allergies. It calms and rejuvenates your nervous system.

Nadi Shodhana helps balance your hormones, aids mental clarity, and enhances concentration. It equalizes the right and left hemispheres of your brain, and your masculine-solar, and feminine-lunar, energies.

Kapalabhati – Shining Skull Breath*

Kapalabhati comes from two Sanskrit words: *Kapala* = "skull" and *Bhati* = "light." When practicing *Kapalabhati*, many yogis experience a sensation of either literal light, or a feeling of lightness.

How to Create Kapalabhati Breath

Sit in a comfortable position with your hands on your lower belly. Inhale deeply through your nose, and exhale deeply through your nose. Feel your lower belly expand when you inhale and contract when you exhale. This requires that you breathe deeply into the depths of your core.

Inhale again and then exhale, contracting your lower belly sharply, with the breath forced out in a short burst. You will see your hands move in and out on your belly.

After the sharp exhale, your body will naturally inhale, passively. The attention is to the sharp, deep belly exhale. Keep your spine and shoulders still, the only movement is in your lower belly. Do this 20 times and pause, checking in with your body.

When first practicing *Kapalabhati* you may experience lightheadedness, or a slight dizziness. Progress slowly if you experience these symptoms, but the goal is to get up to 75 or 100 repetitions. If you feel dizzy or become anxious, or your breath becomes strained, stop and breathe calmly.

Do the *Kapalabhati* breathing for no longer than a minute, then breathe deeply and exhale slowly as you calm into the quiet *Kapalabhati* produces.

Kapalabhati Breath and Your Health

Kapalabhati is invigorating and warming. It tones and cleanses your lungs, sinuses, and your respiratory system by stimulating the release of toxins, while refreshing and rejuvenating your body, mind, and spirit.

Practiced regularly, *Kapalabhati* will strengthen your diaphragm and abdominal muscles. It increases your body's oxygen supply thus stimulating your brain, even as it calms the mind for meditation, or work that requires strong focus.

With practice, you will discover that *Kapalabhati*—and all yoga breathing exercises—brings balance into your life on physical, mental, emotional, and spiritual levels.

*Kapalabhati is counter-indicated for people with high blood pressure, a hernia, or heart disease. Practice conservatively if you have asthma or emphysema, and stop if you're experiencing discomfort. The goal is to become more relaxed, and any breath exercise that generates tension is counterproductive to that goal.

Breath is the blossoming
of each moment.
Be in the moment.
Blythe Ayne

Favorite Yoga Routines

One of the many wonderful aspects of yoga is that you can make it yours in any way that suits you best. Here you can write down sequences you've developed that let you completely relax, that empower you, that strengthen your body, that enhance your mind, and nurture your spirit.

A Favorite Restorative Routine:

_____

_____

_____

_____

_____

_____

_____

_____

_____

_____

_____

_____

_____

_____

_____

_____

_____

_____

_____

A Favorite Restorative Routine:

_____
_____
_____
_____
_____
_____
_____
_____
_____
_____
_____
_____
_____
_____
_____
_____
_____
_____
_____
_____
_____
_____
_____
_____

A Favorite Rejuvenating Routine:

A Favorite Rejuvenating Routine:

_____

_____

_____

_____

_____

_____

_____

_____

_____

_____

_____

_____

_____

_____

_____

_____

_____

_____

_____

_____

_____

_____

_____

_____

_____

_____

My Gift for You ....

Download your copy of
Save Your Life with Stupendous Spices
at: bit.ly/SpicesBookFunnel

You'll also receive my occasional newsletter, *Your Amazing Life*, with interesting info about Body, Mind, and Spirit for your happy, healthy life.

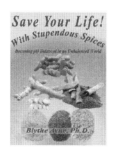

About the Author

I live in a forest with a few domestic and numerous wild creatures, where I create an ever-growing inventory of books, both nonfiction and fiction, short stories, illustrated kid's books, and articles, with a bit of wood carving when I need a change of pace. I've practiced yoga for decades with amazing teachers, always keeping for myself a beginner, no competition, mindset.

I received my Doctorate from the University of California at Irvine in the School of Social Sciences, majoring in psychology and ethnography, after which I moved to the Pacific Northwest to write and to have a modest private psychotherapy practice in a small town not much bigger than a village. Finally I decided it was time to put my full focus on my writing, where, through the world-shrinking internet, I could "meet" greater numbers of people. *Where I could meet you!*

All the creatures in my forest and I thank you for "stopping by" and sharing some quiet, healing yoga.

I Wish You Happiness, Health, Peace, and Joy,
Blythe

Questions, comments? I'd love to hear from you!:

Blythe@BlytheAyne.com

www.BlytheAyne.com

Printed in Great Britain
by Amazon